RIDE THE BLACK HORSE

NICK WARD

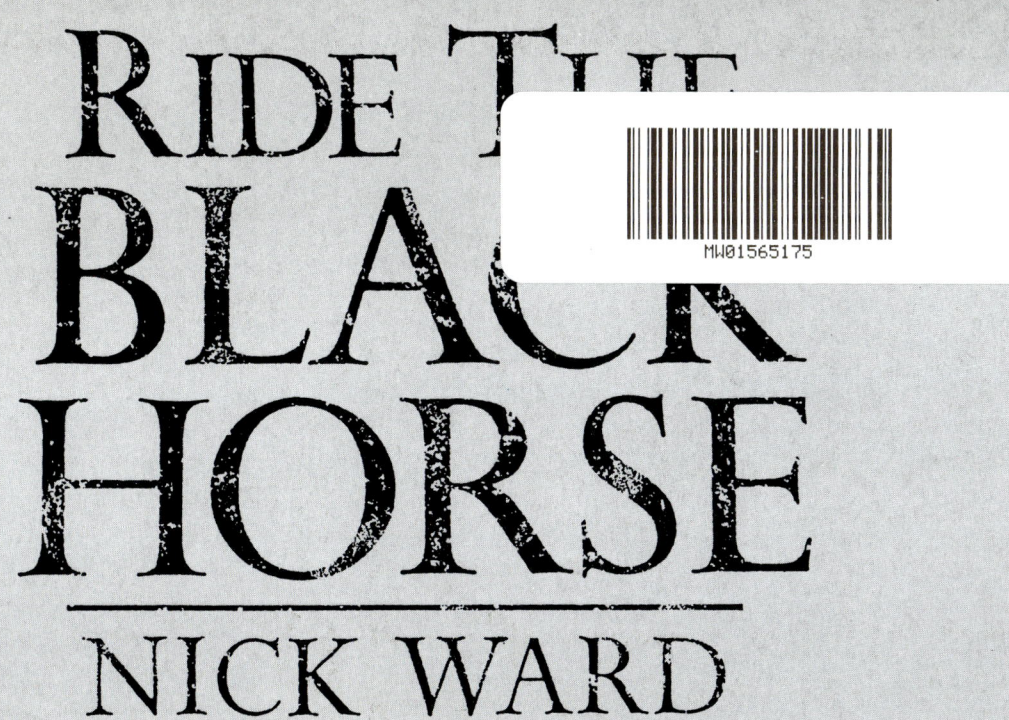

OXFORD UNIVERSITY PRESS

OXFORD TORONTO MELBOURNE

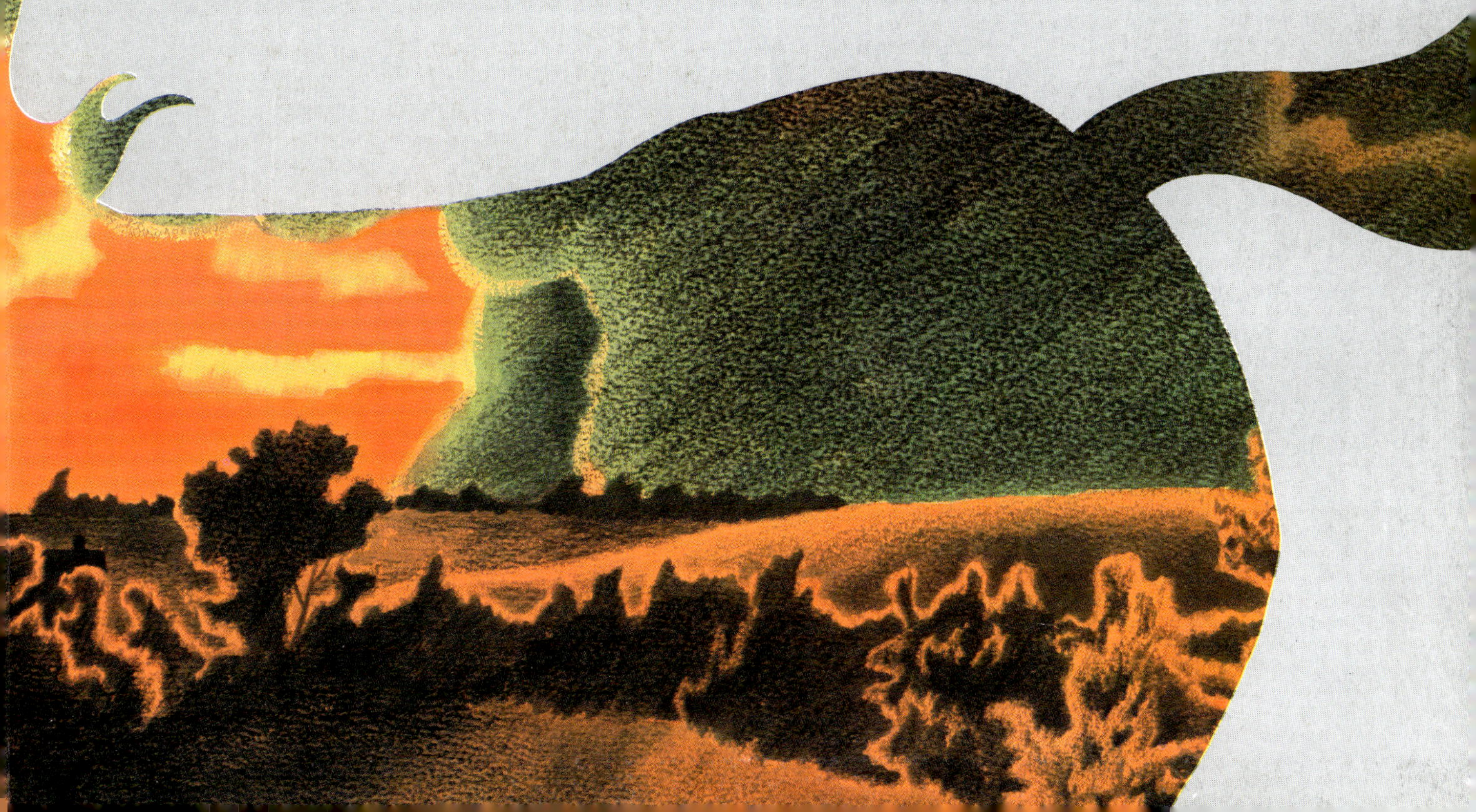

Oxford University Press, Walton Street, Oxford OX2 6DP

Oxford New York Toronto
Kuala Lumpur Singapore Hong Kong Tokyo
Delhi Bombay Calcutta Madras Karachi
Nairobi Dar es Salaam Cape Town
Melbourne Auckland

and associated companies in
Beirut Berlin Ibadan Mexico City Nicosia

Oxford is a trade mark of Oxford University Press

© Nick Ward 1986
First published 1986

All rights reserved. No part of this publication may be reproduced,
stored in a retrieval system, or transmitted, in any form, or by any means
electronic, mechanical, photocopying, recording, or otherwise, without the
prior permission of Oxford University Press

This book is sold subject to the condition that it shall not, by way of
trade or otherwise, be lent, re-sold, hired or otherwise circulated,
without the publisher's prior consent in any form of binding or cover
other than that in which it is published and without a similar condition
including this condition being imposed on the subsequent purchaser

British Library Cataloguing in Publication Data
Ward, Nick
  Ride the black horse.
  I. Title
  823'.914[J]   PZ7
  ISBN 0–19–279806–5

Typeset by Oxford Publishing Services, Oxford
Printed in Hong Kong

For Nick Brennan

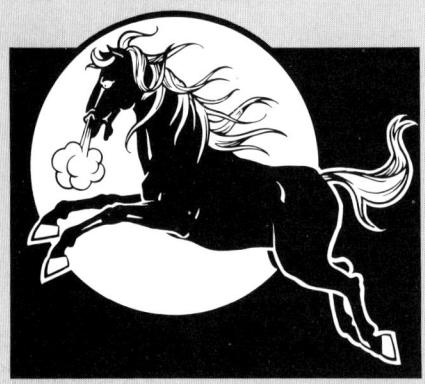

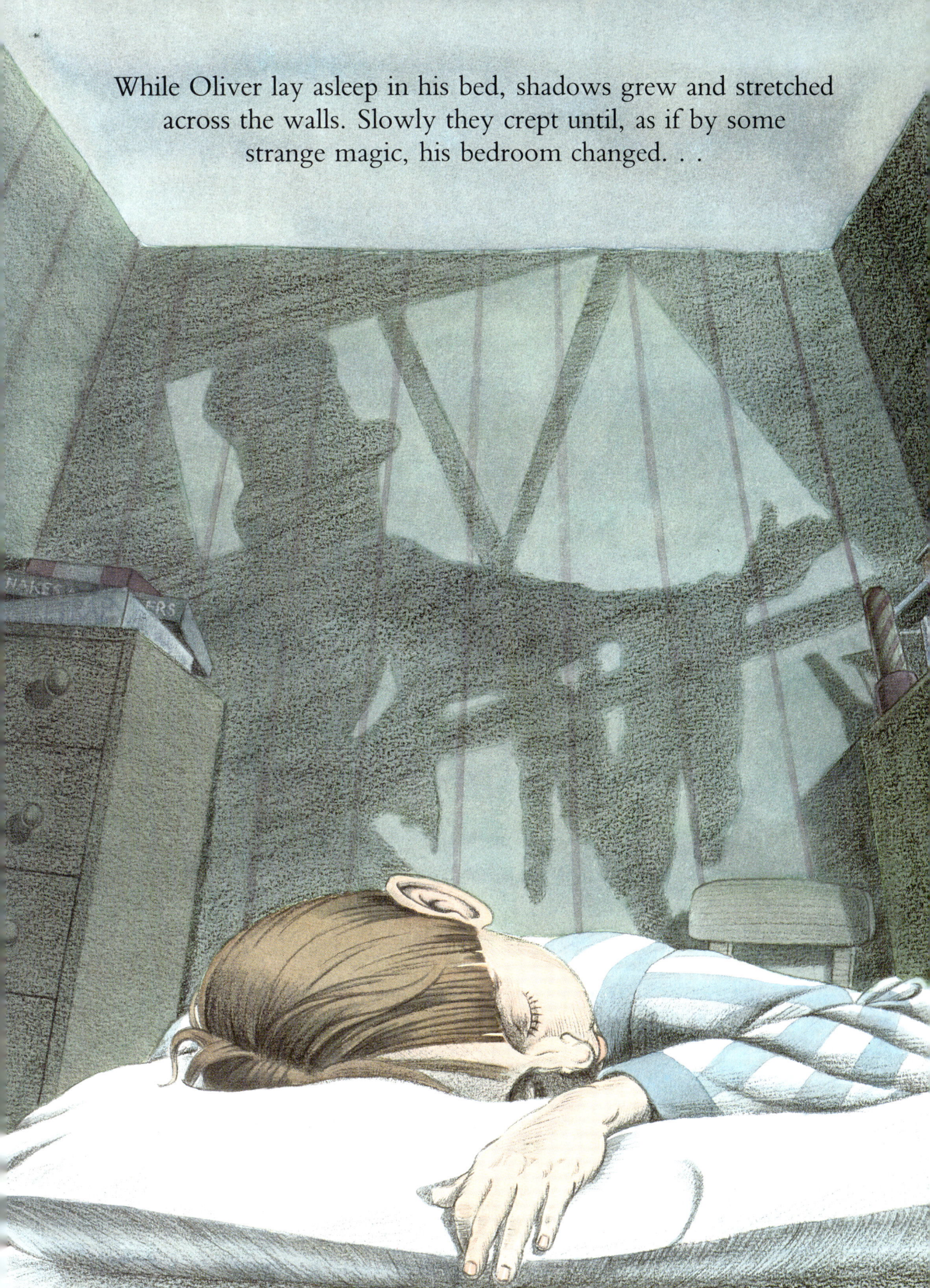

While Oliver lay asleep in his bed, shadows grew and stretched across the walls. Slowly they crept until, as if by some strange magic, his bedroom changed...

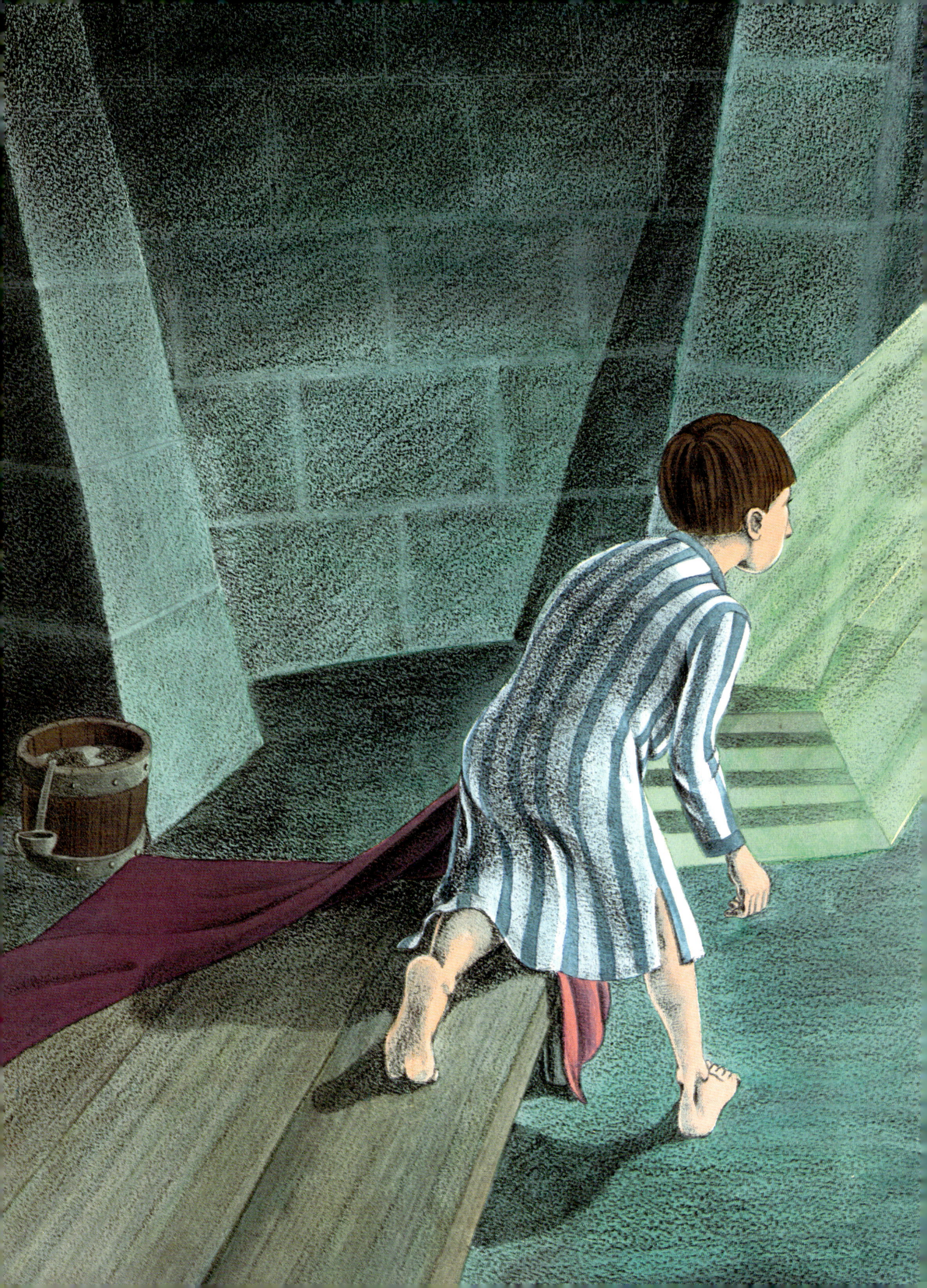

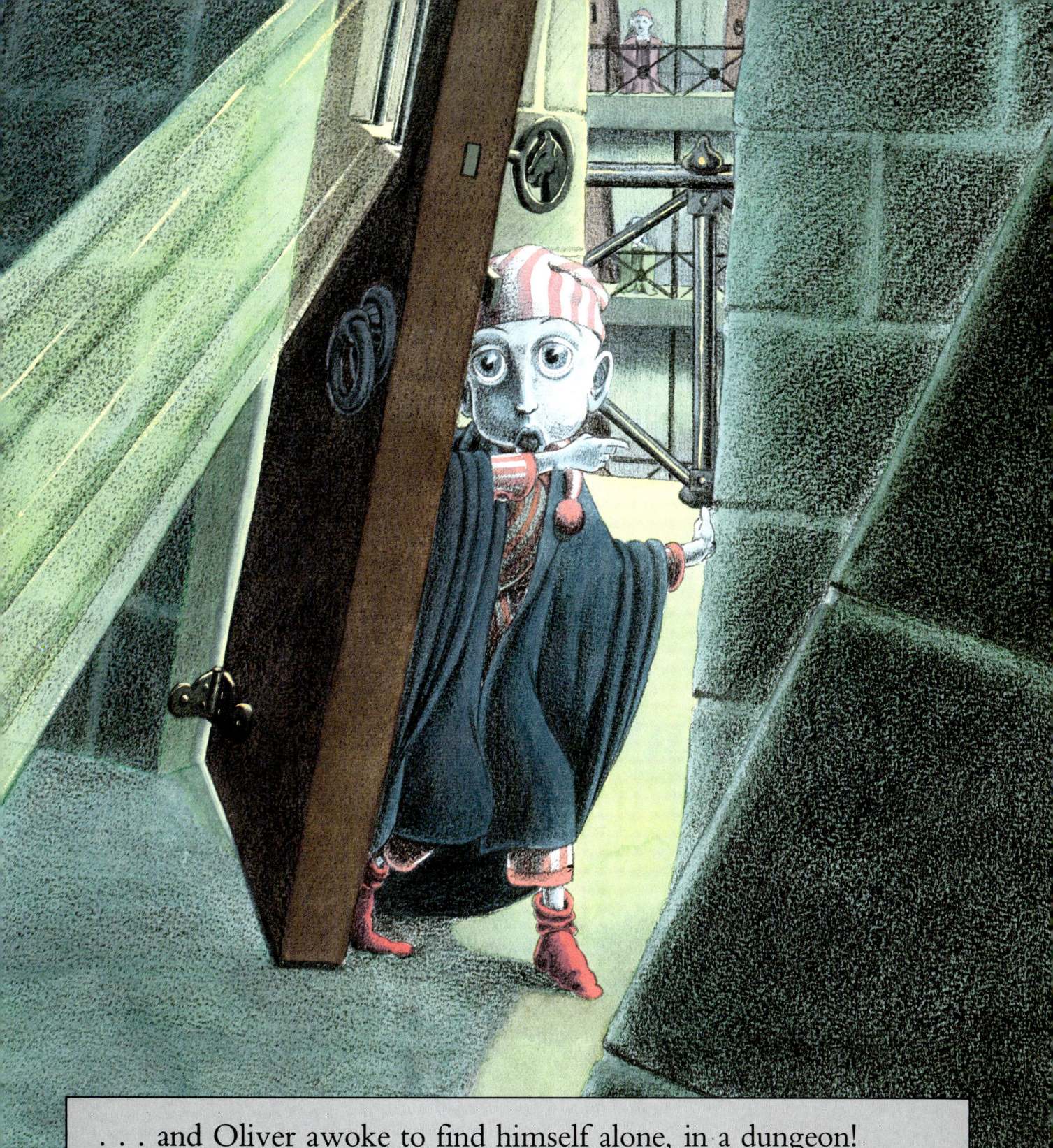

. . . and Oliver awoke to find himself alone, in a dungeon!

He heard a key turning, and a heavy door creaked open. A small, frightened creature peered in.
'What is the meaning of this,' demanded Oliver. 'Where am I?'
'No time for questions,' squeaked the creature in reply. 'There is to be a show just for you!'

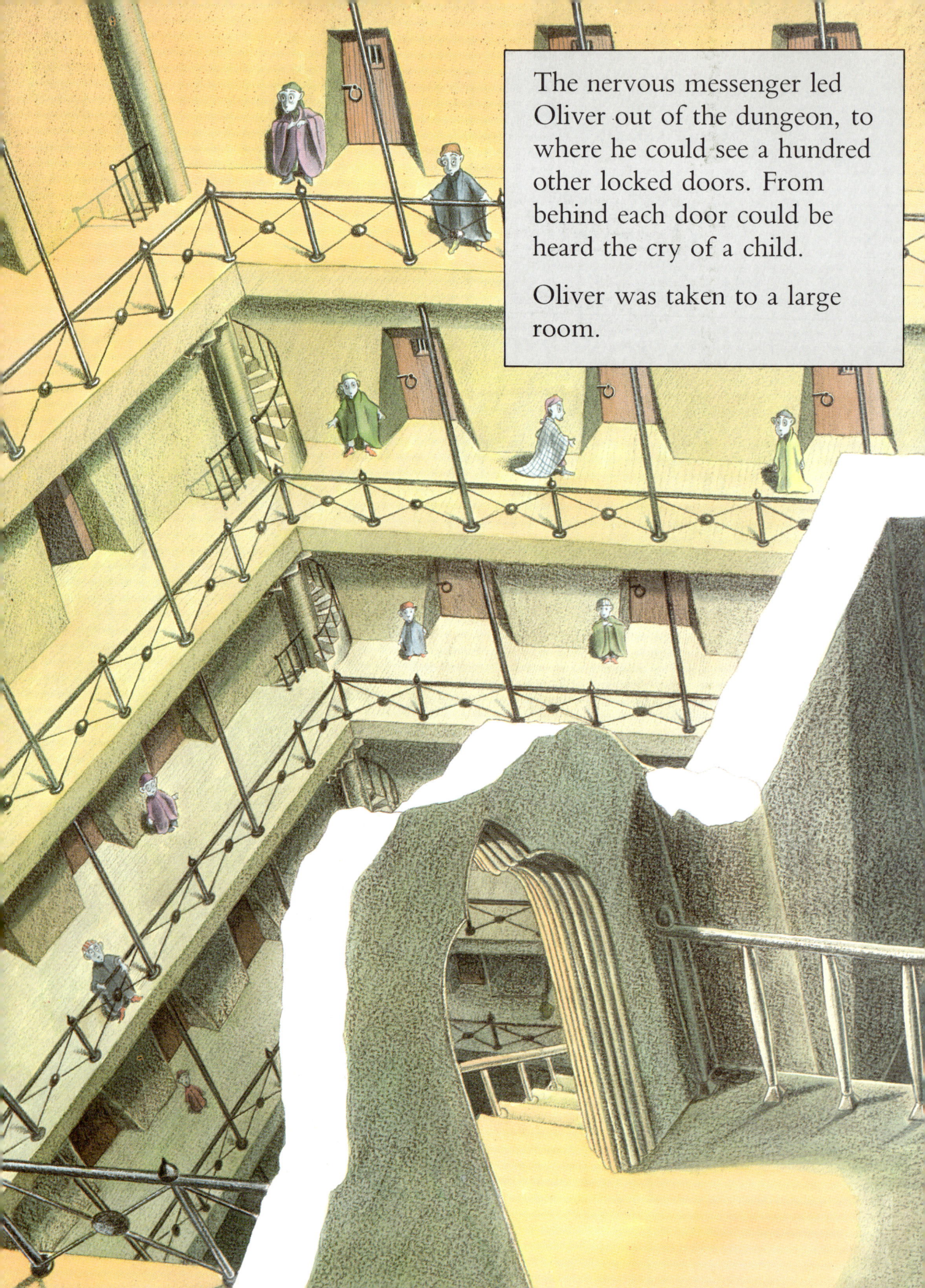

The nervous messenger led Oliver out of the dungeon, to where he could see a hundred other locked doors. From behind each door could be heard the cry of a child.

Oliver was taken to a large room.

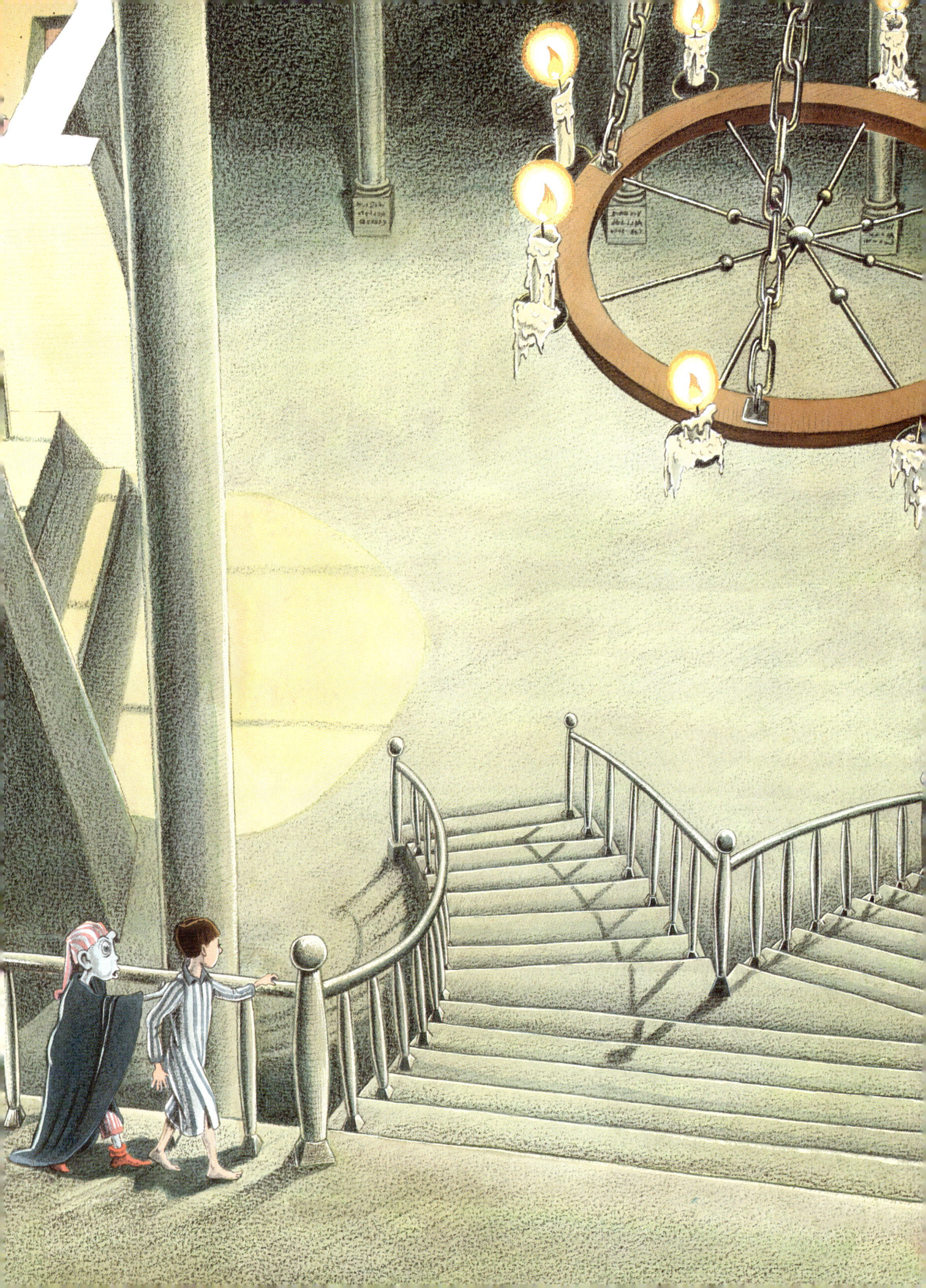

In the darkest corner, the blackest shadow shook itself free, and grew, shaping itself to become a most awesome magician. 'Welcome to my show,' he whispered.

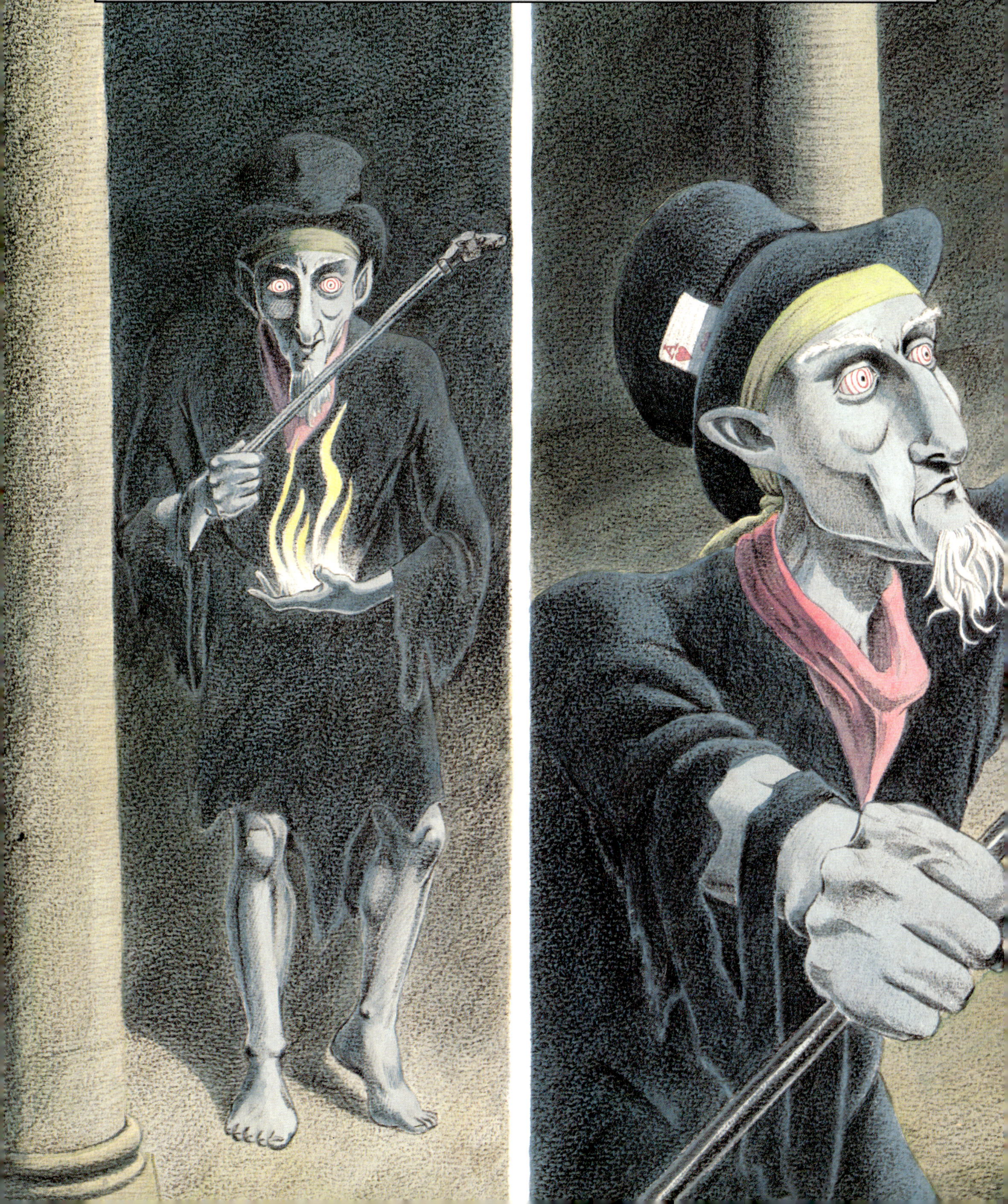

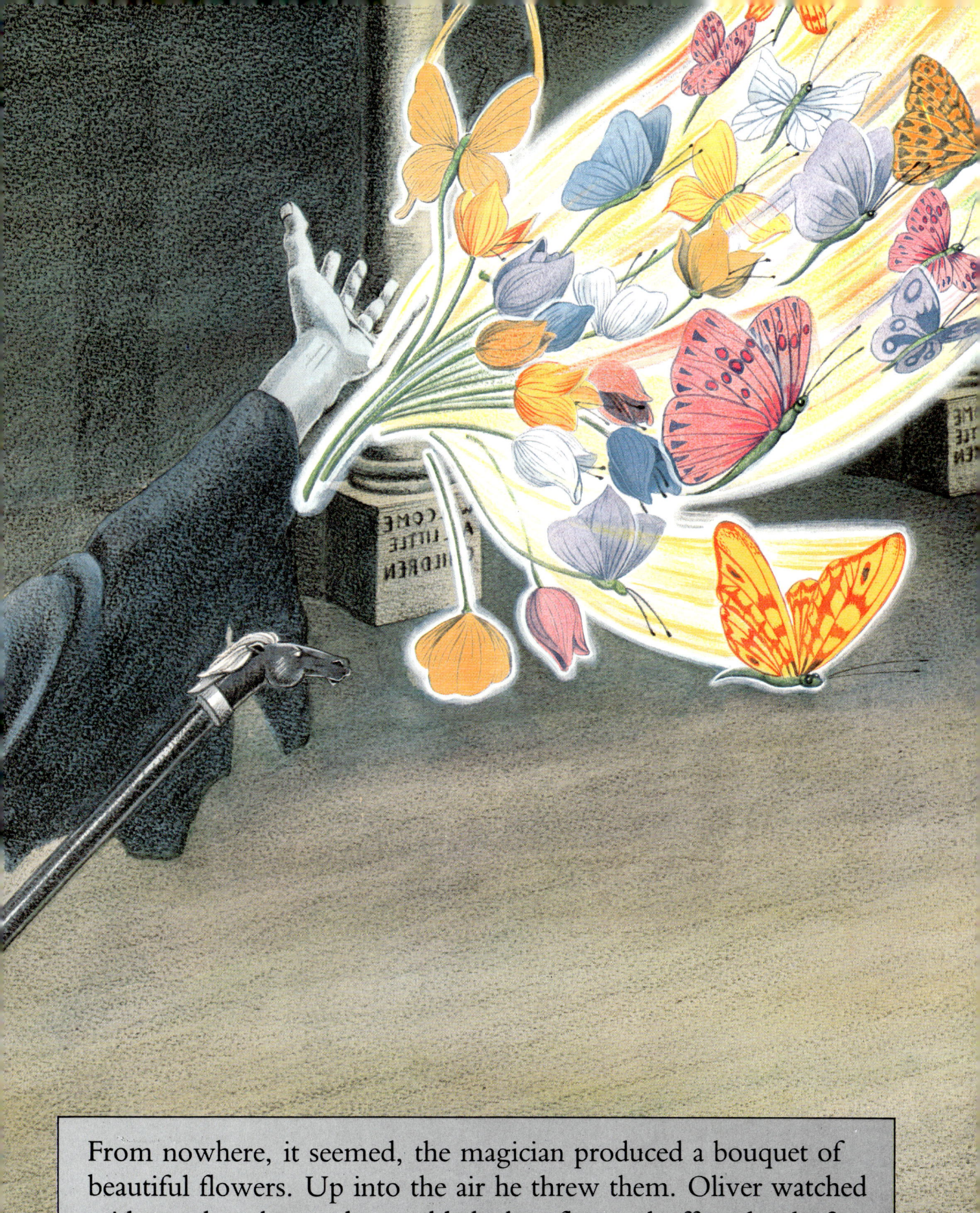

From nowhere, it seemed, the magician produced a bouquet of beautiful flowers. Up into the air he threw them. Oliver watched wide-eyed as the petals trembled, then fluttered off, a cloud of coloured butterflies.

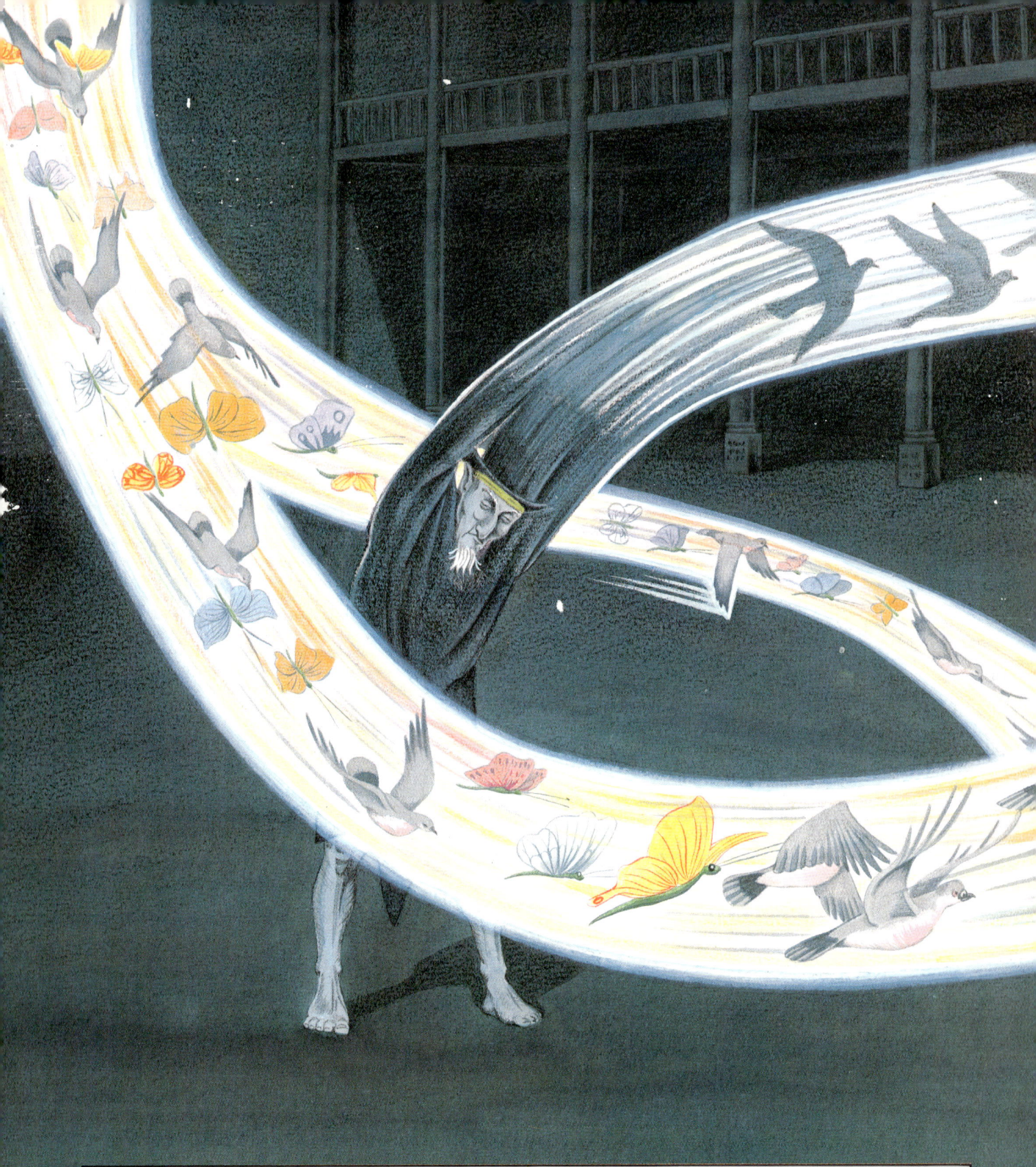

He stared in wonder as the magician himself began to shudder, then broke into a flock of calling birds that flew up to join the butterflies.

It seemed the whole room was full of flapping, flying shapes.

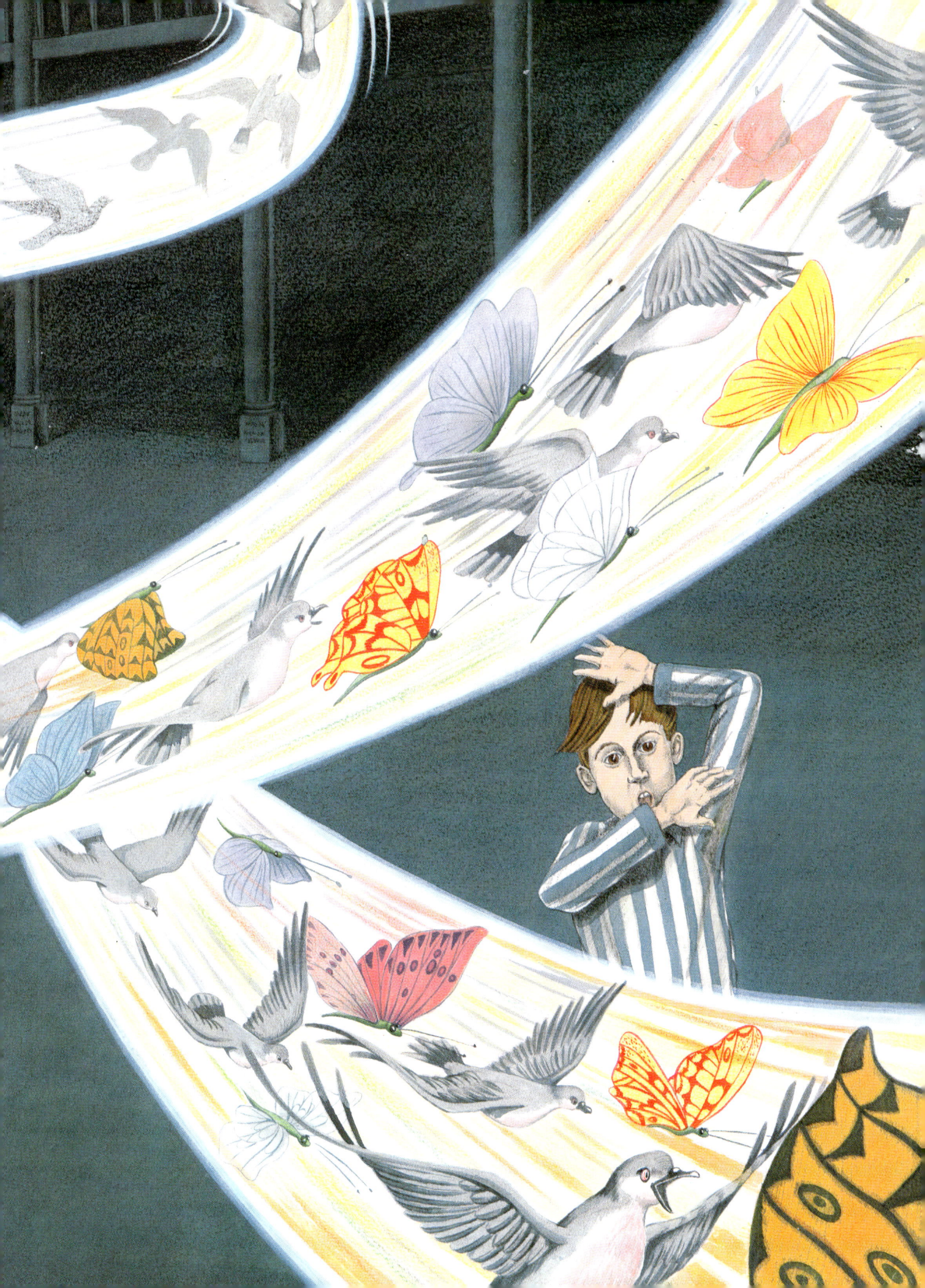

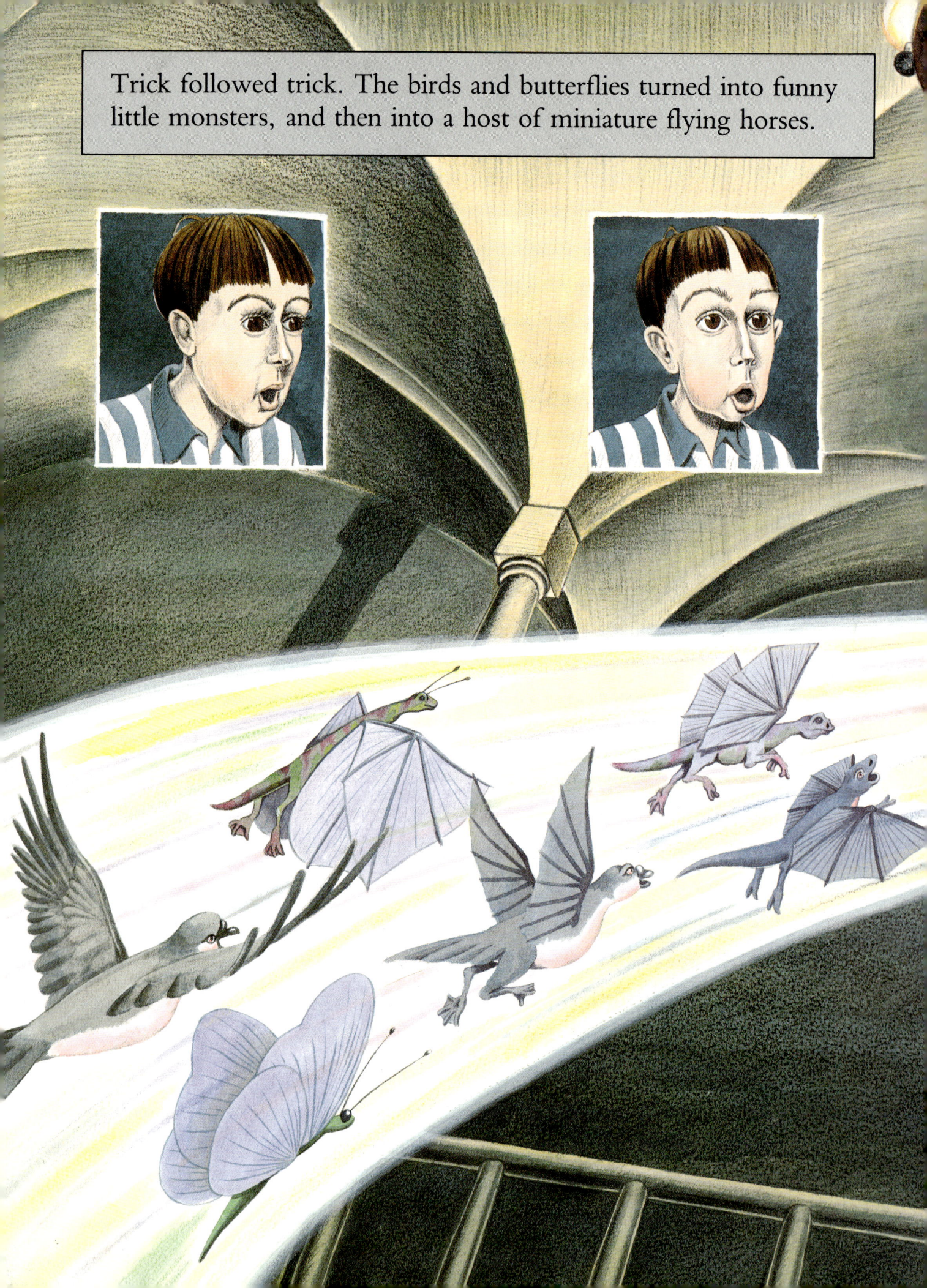

Trick followed trick. The birds and butterflies turned into funny little monsters, and then into a host of miniature flying horses.

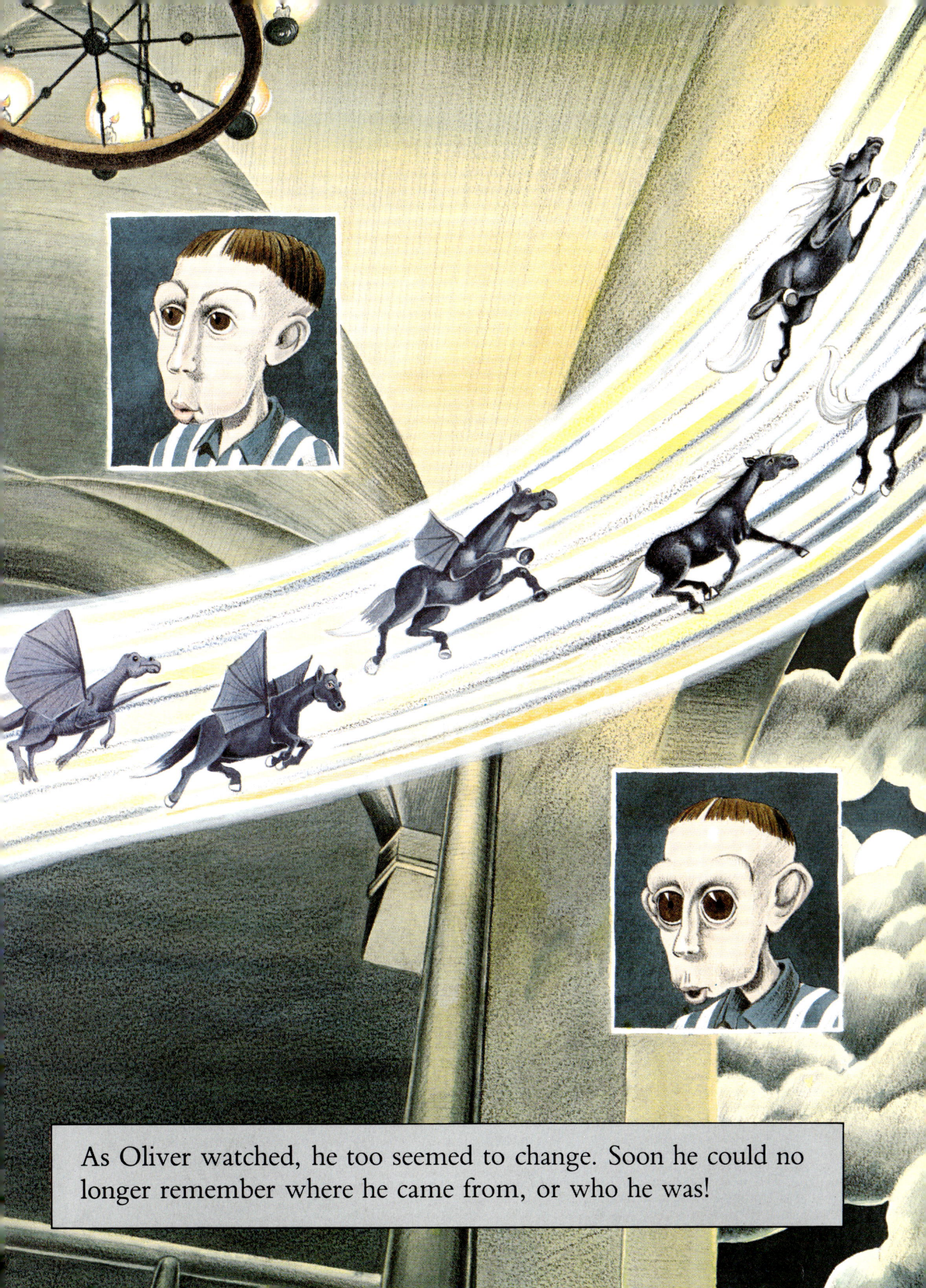

As Oliver watched, he too seemed to change. Soon he could no longer remember where he came from, or who he was!

The tiny horses spun so fast, they quickly became one huge black horse. With stamping feet and steaming breath it called, 'Now you are ready for my final trick.'

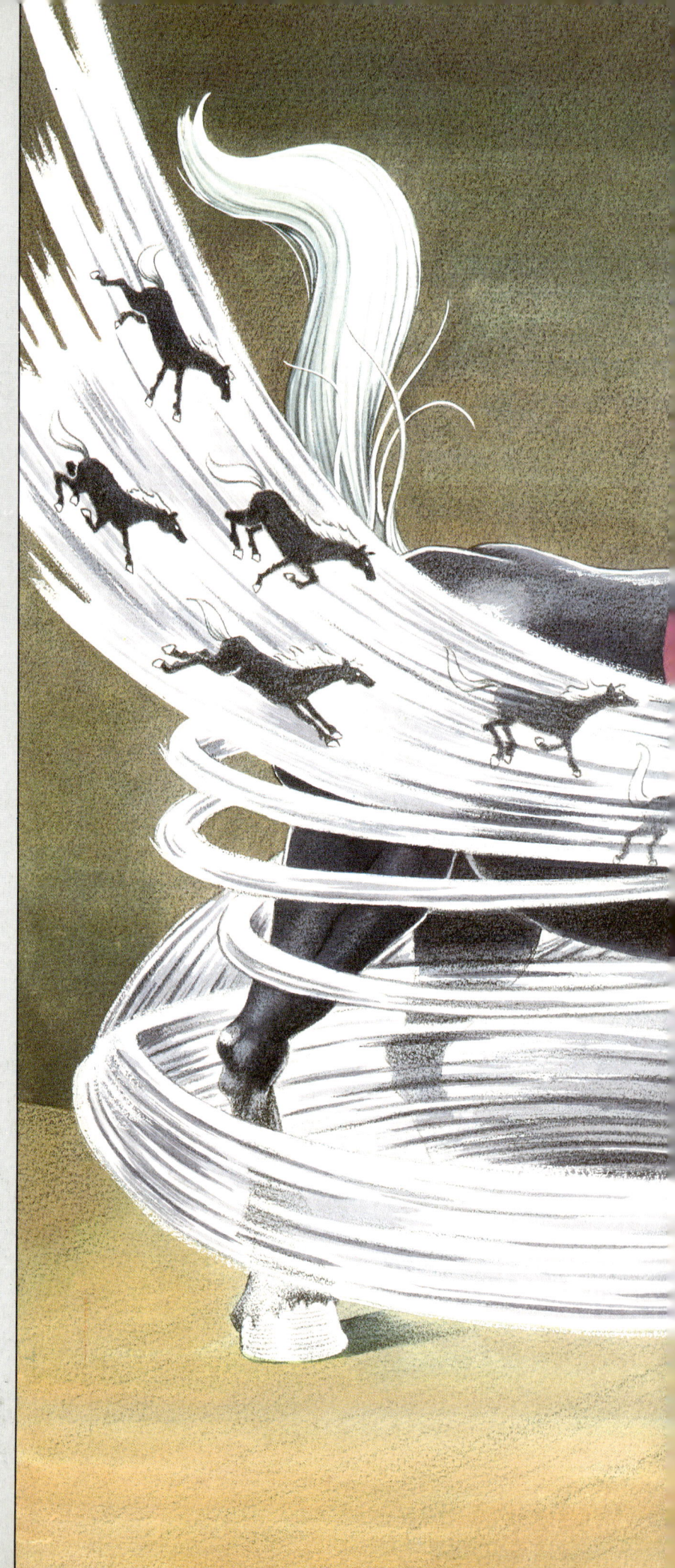

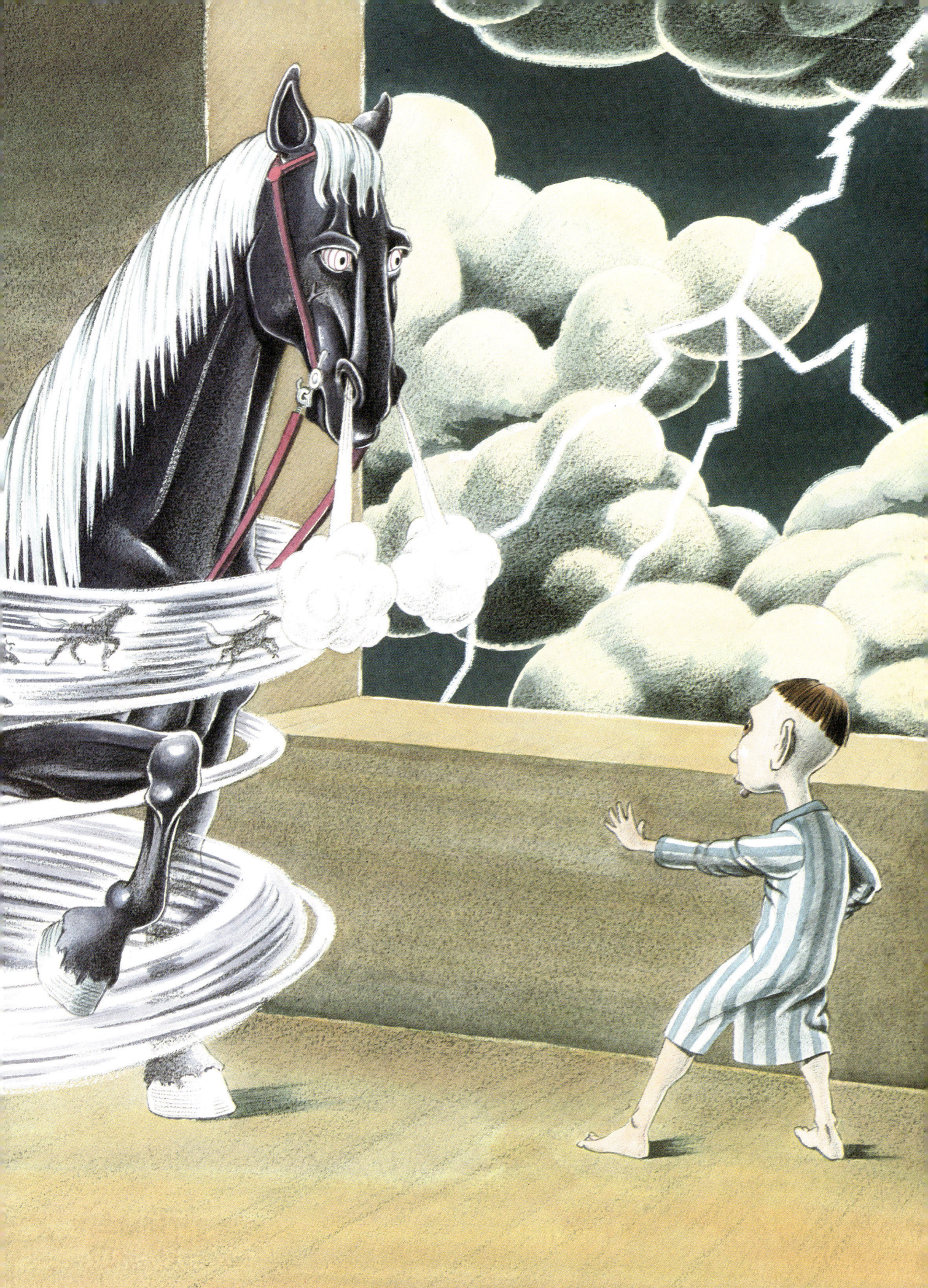

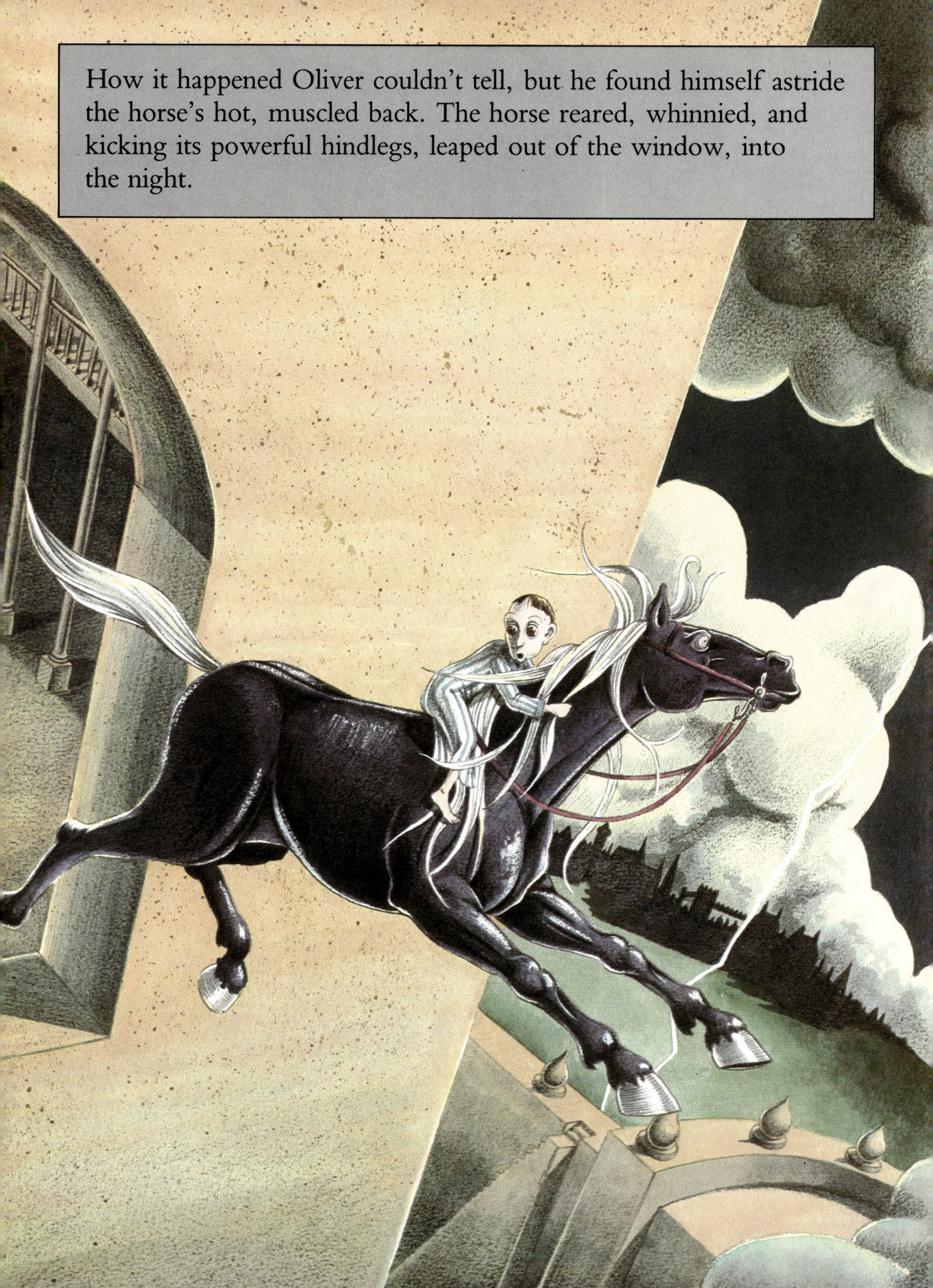

How it happened Oliver couldn't tell, but he found himself astride the horse's hot, muscled back. The horse reared, whinnied, and kicking its powerful hindlegs, leaped out of the window, into the night.

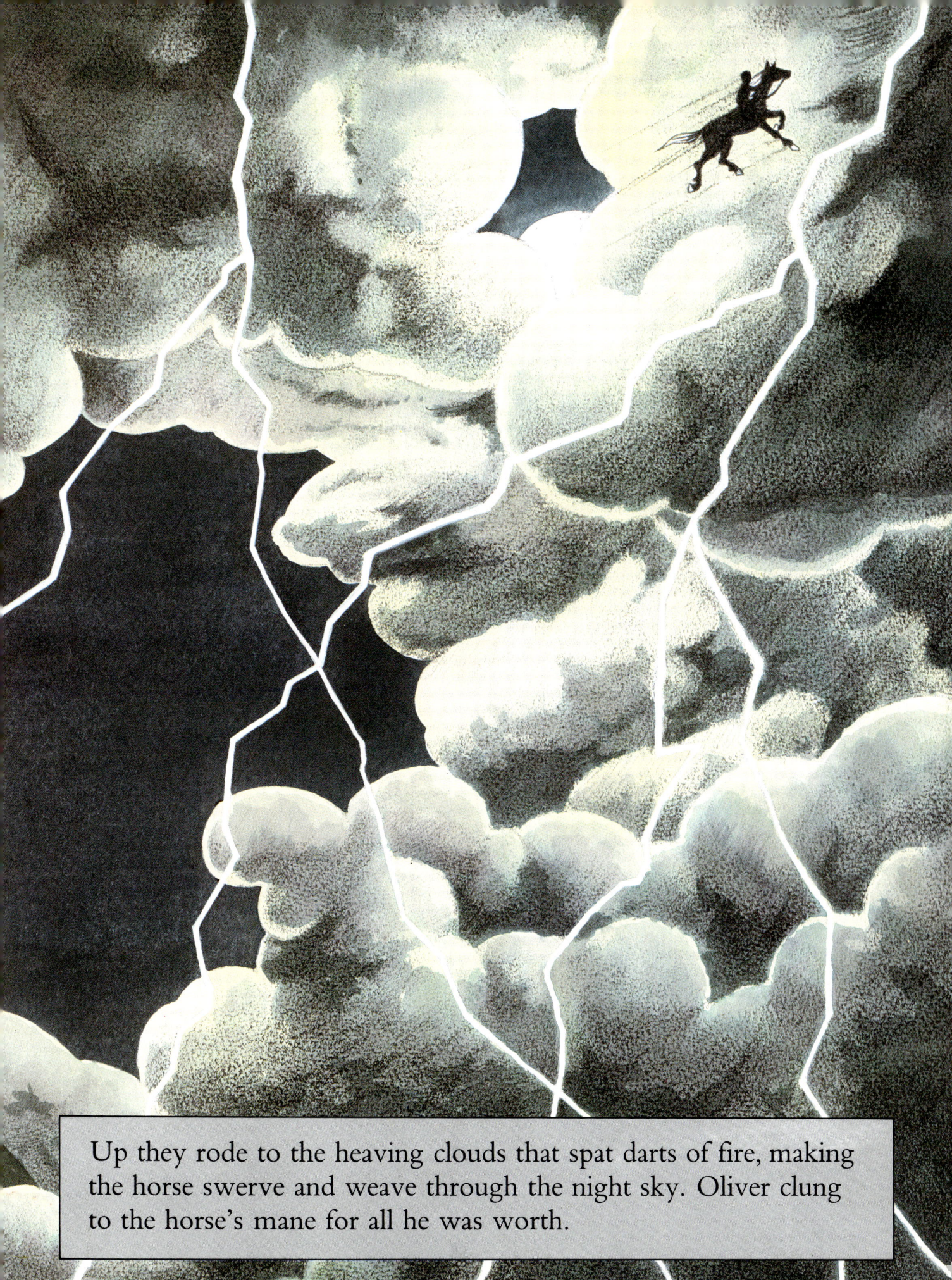

Up they rode to the heaving clouds that spat darts of fire, making the horse swerve and weave through the night sky. Oliver clung to the horse's mane for all he was worth.

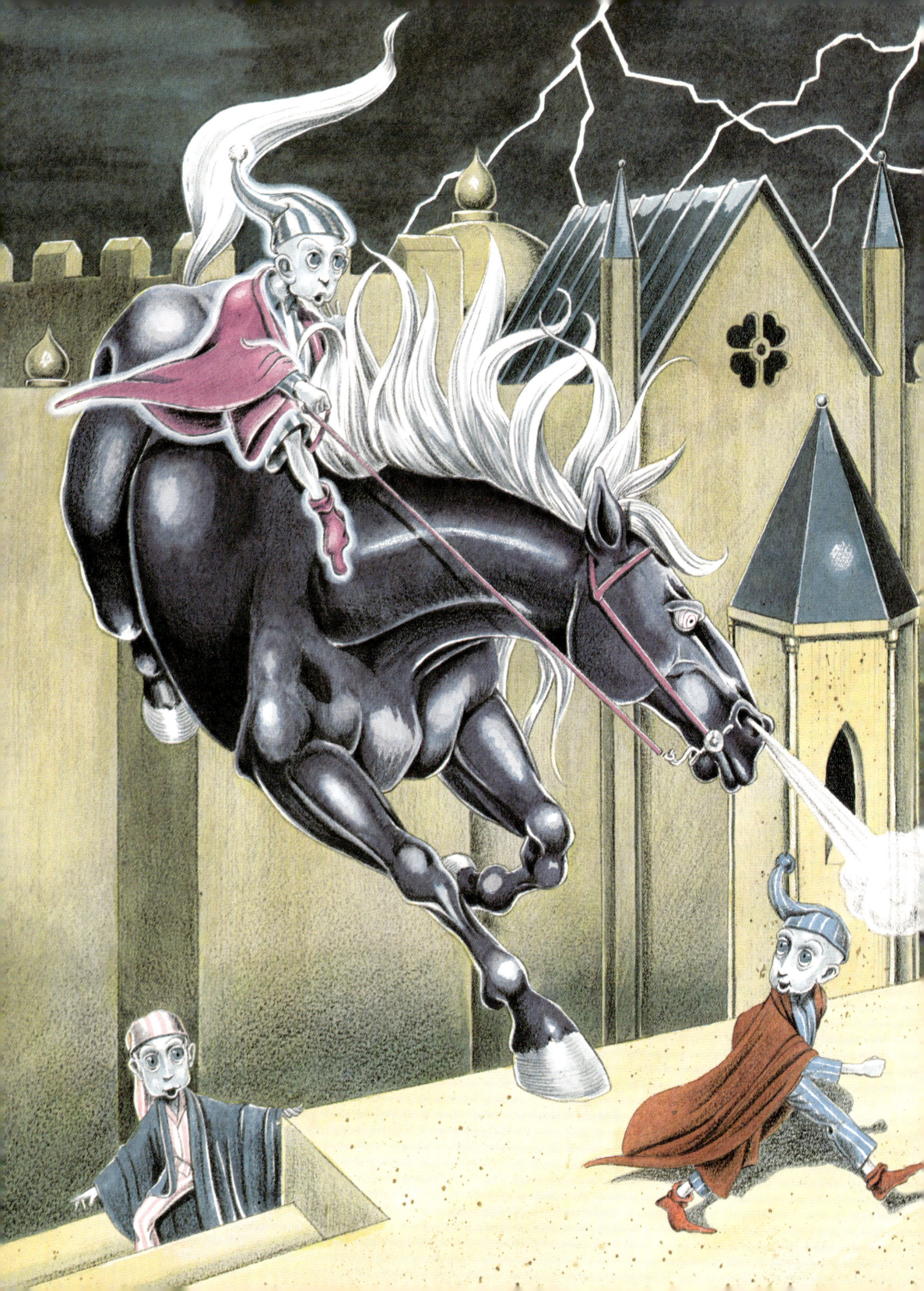

Down they raced, over a crowd of the magician's messengers, who jeered and laughed. This, the magician's final trick, was making Oliver just the same as them! He must do something. . . .

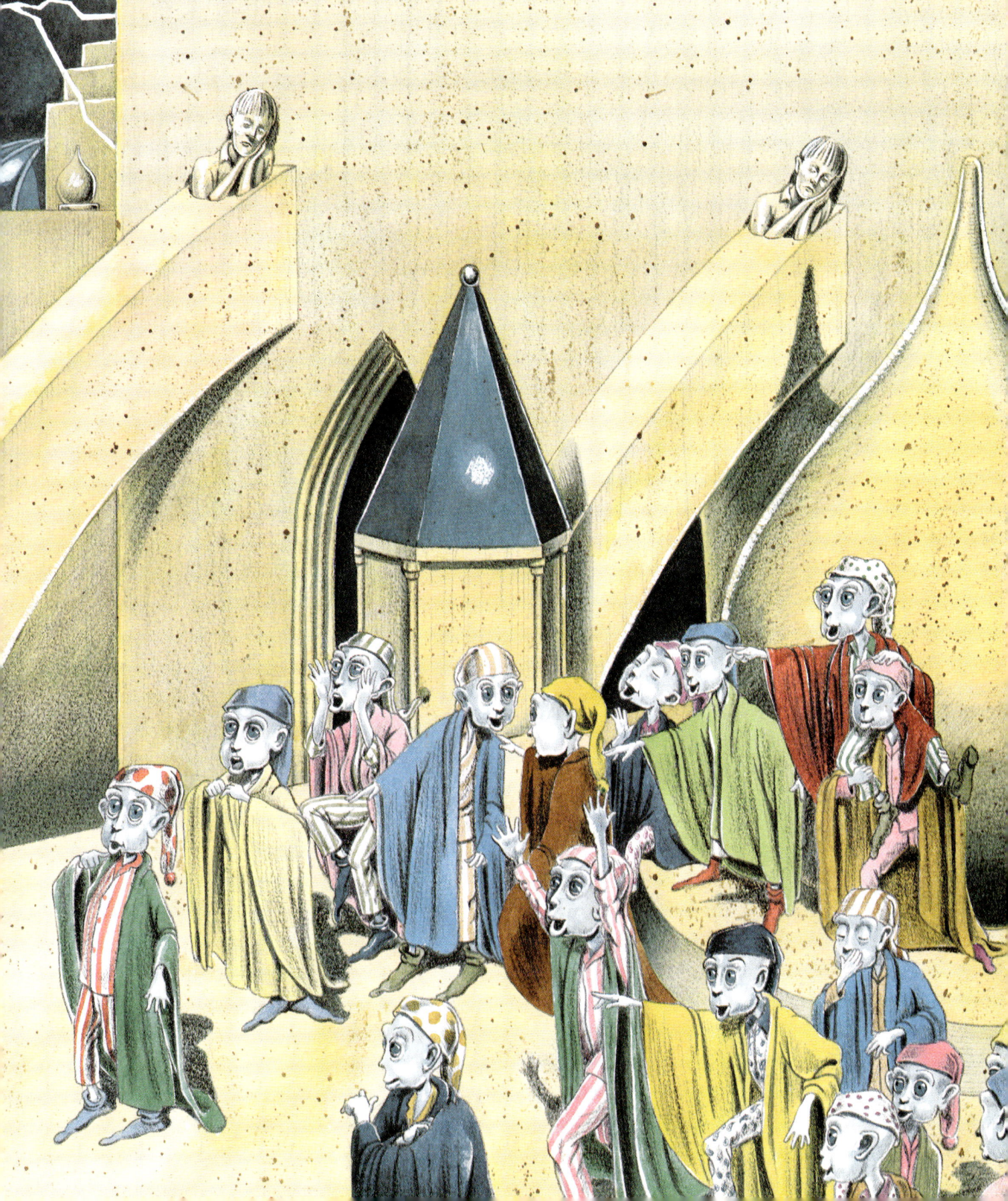

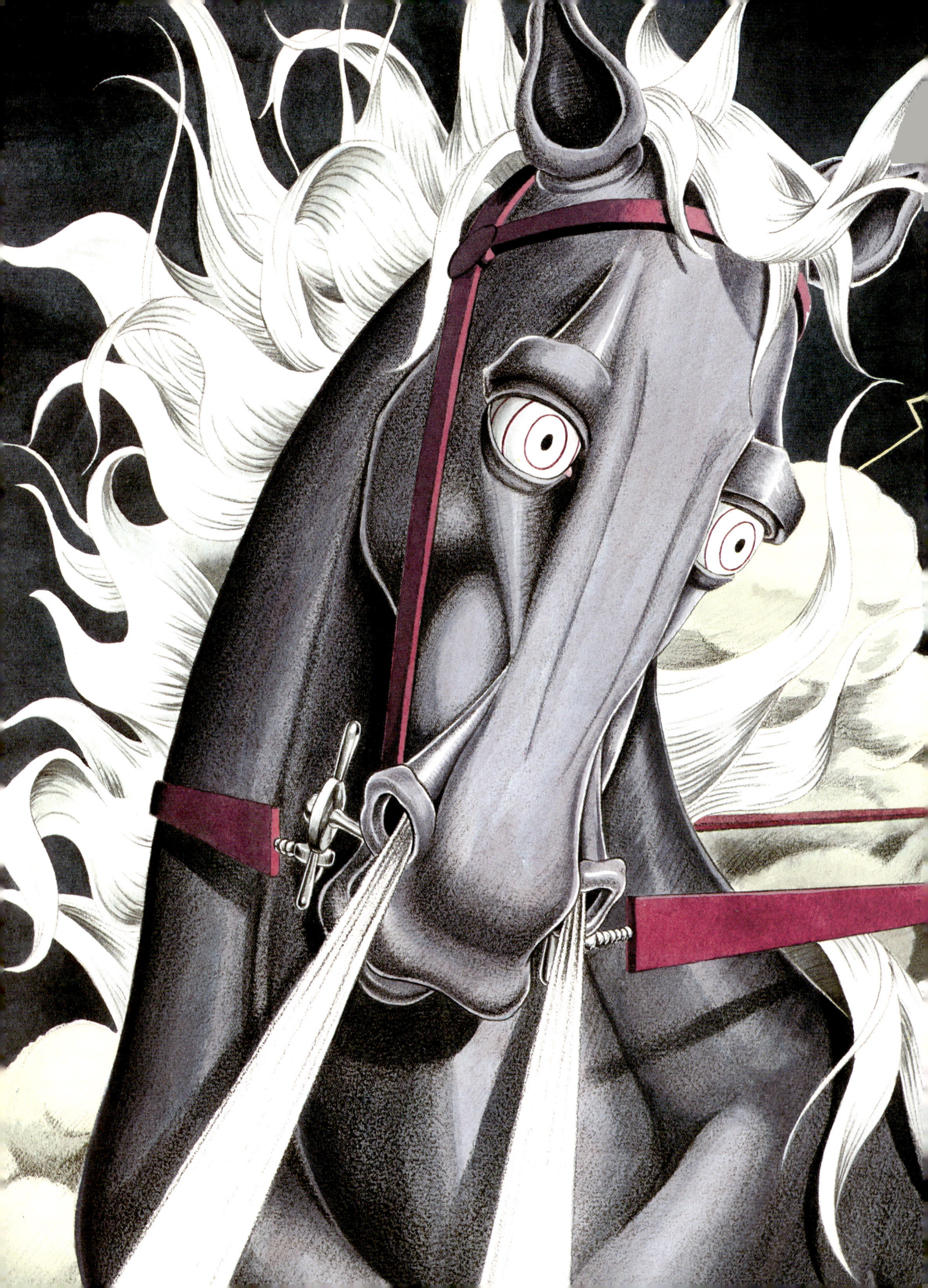

And then Oliver remembered. He remembered his own home, and his own little room. 'I am Oliver,' he shouted. With every bit of strength left in him, he heaved on the reins, until the horse slowed.

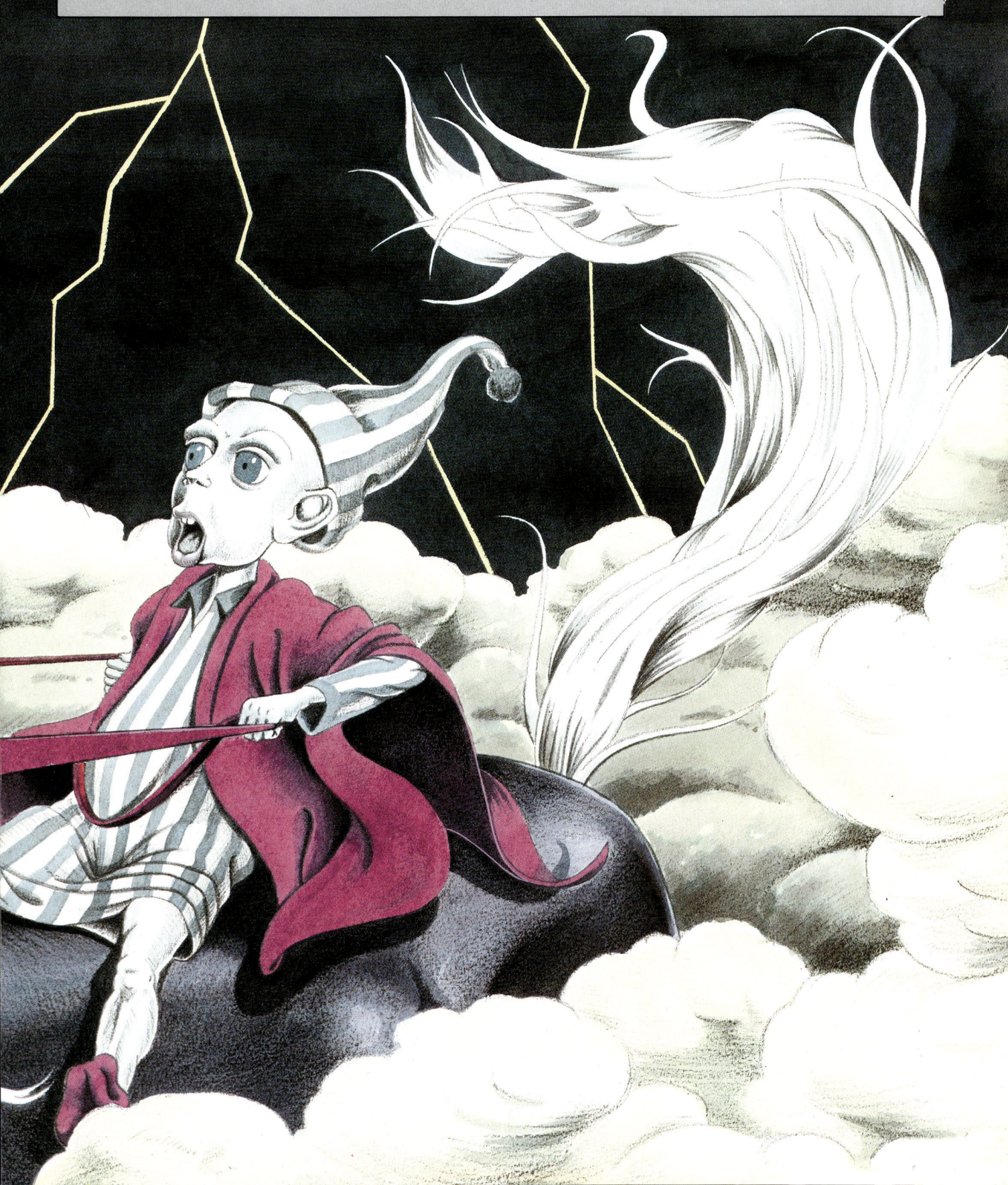

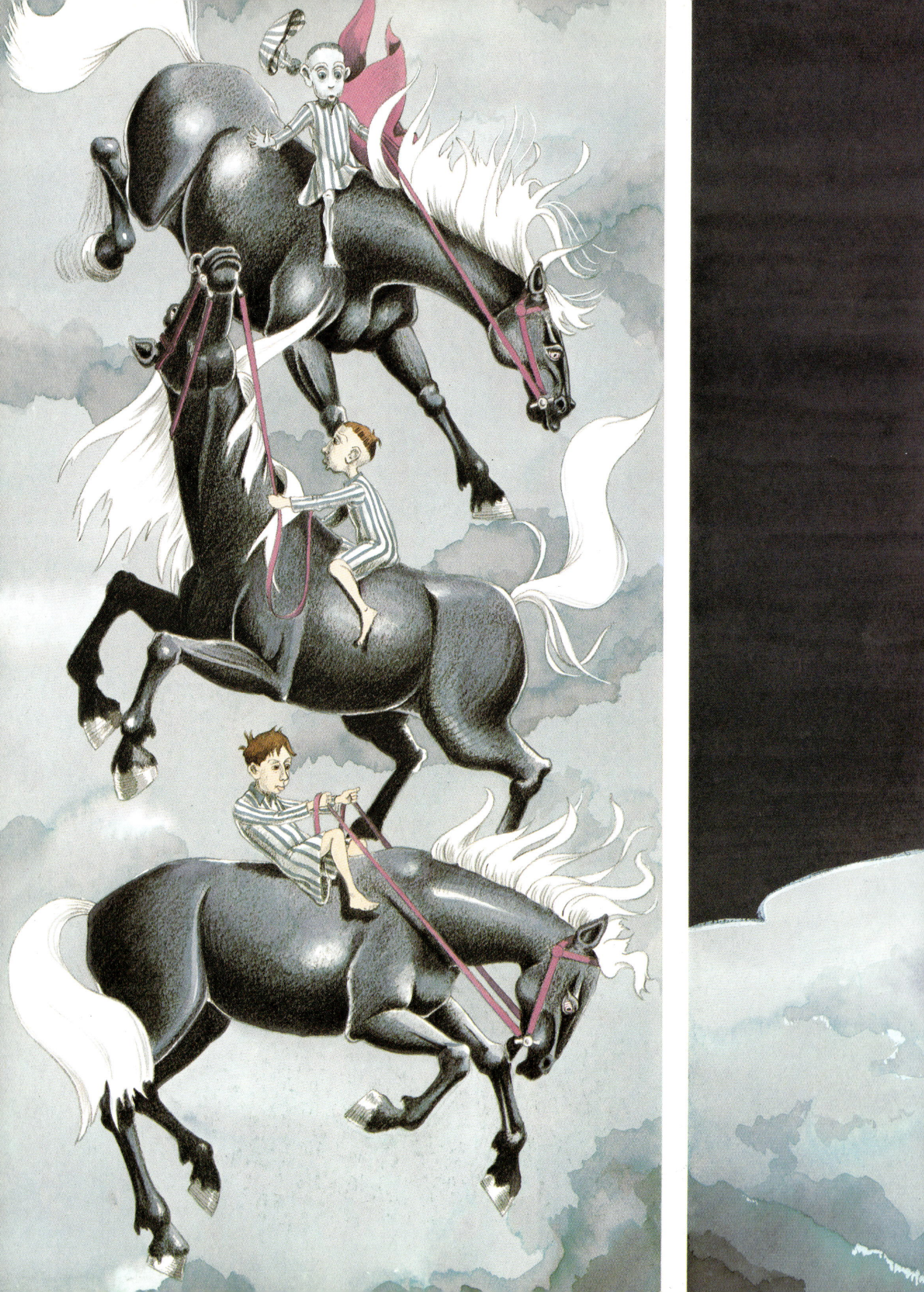

And though the horse kicked and bucked, Oliver would not give in. 'TAKE ME HOME!'

The horse became quiet, then started to melt away from under him, and Oliver became his old self once again.

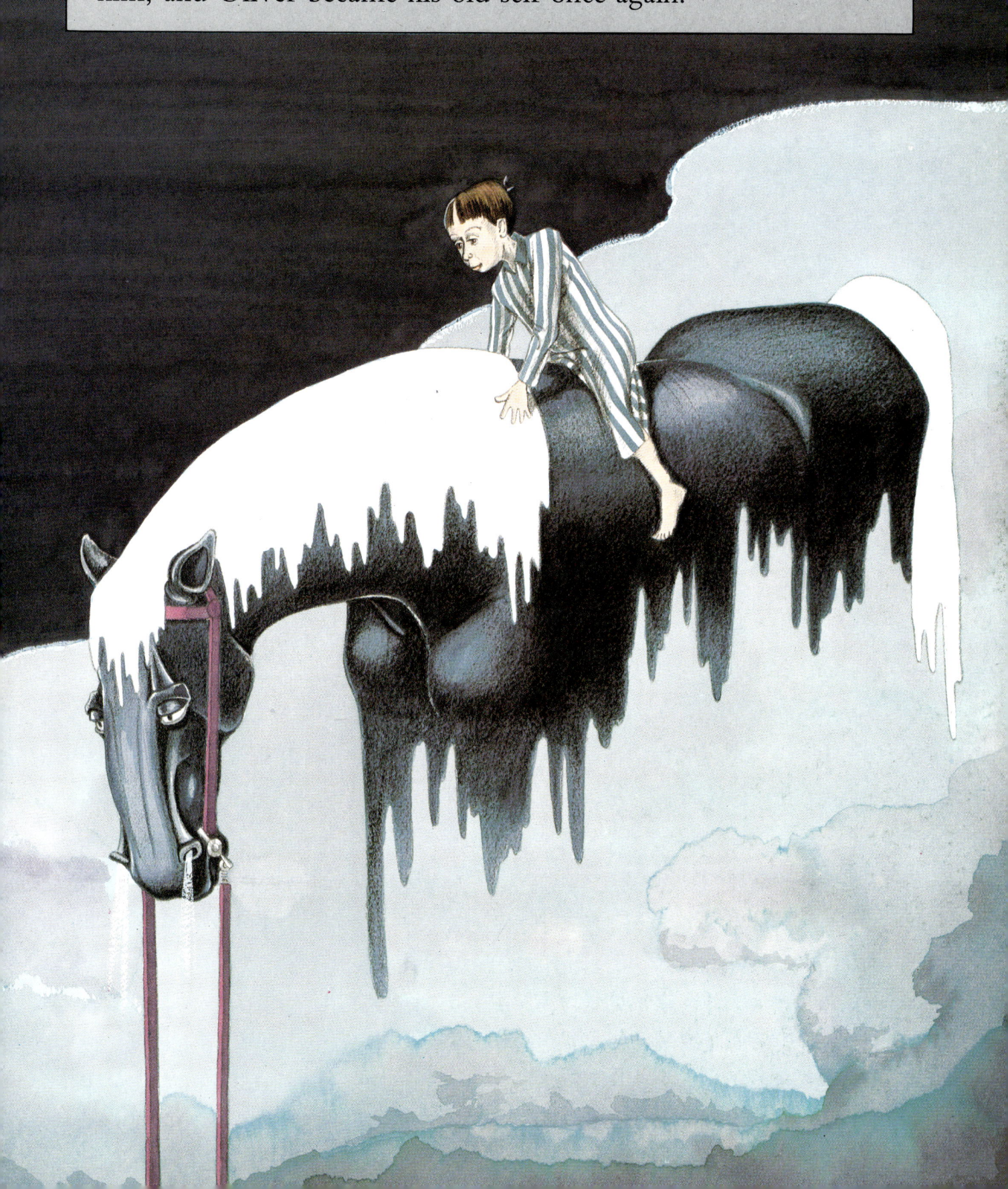

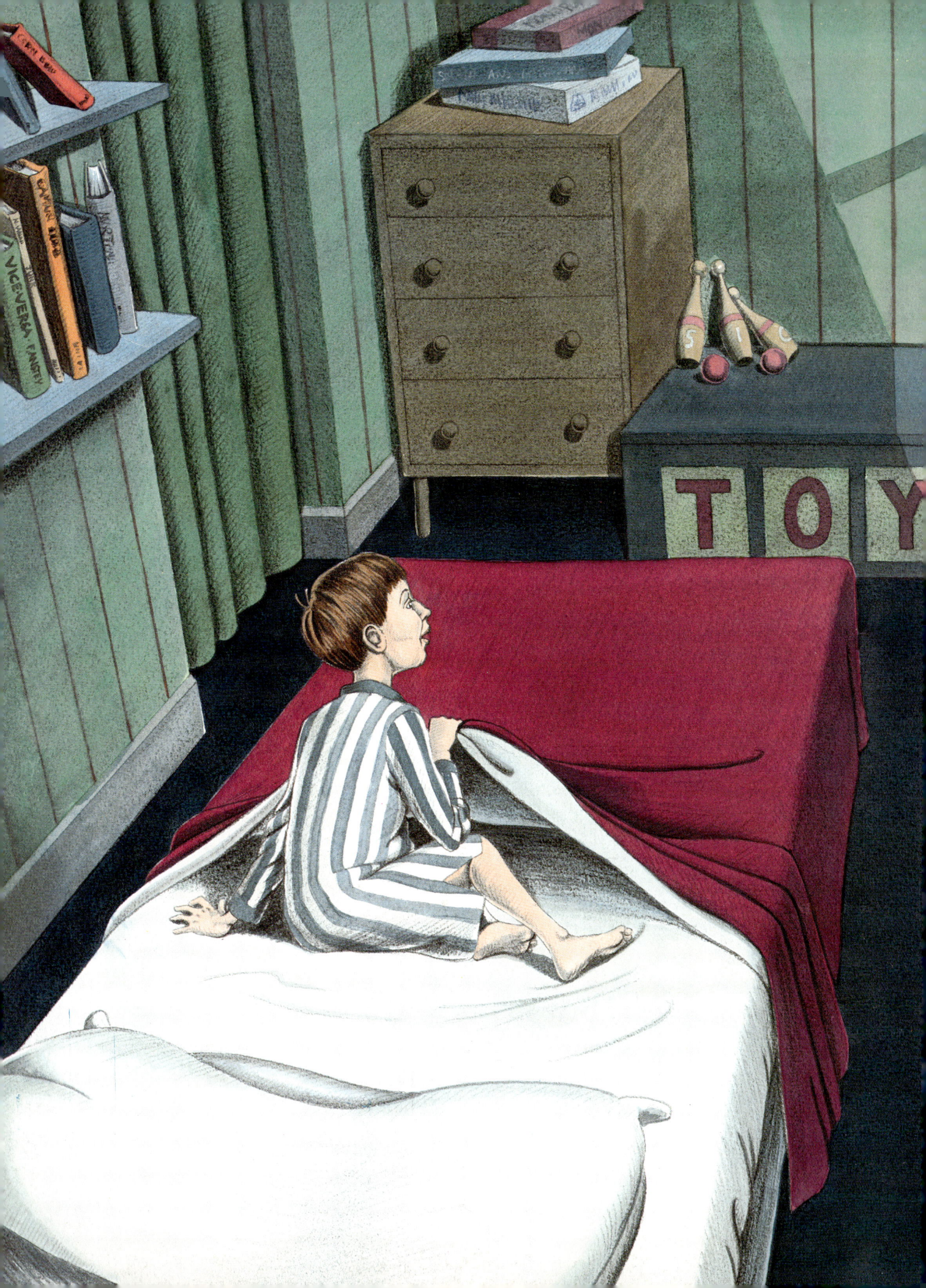

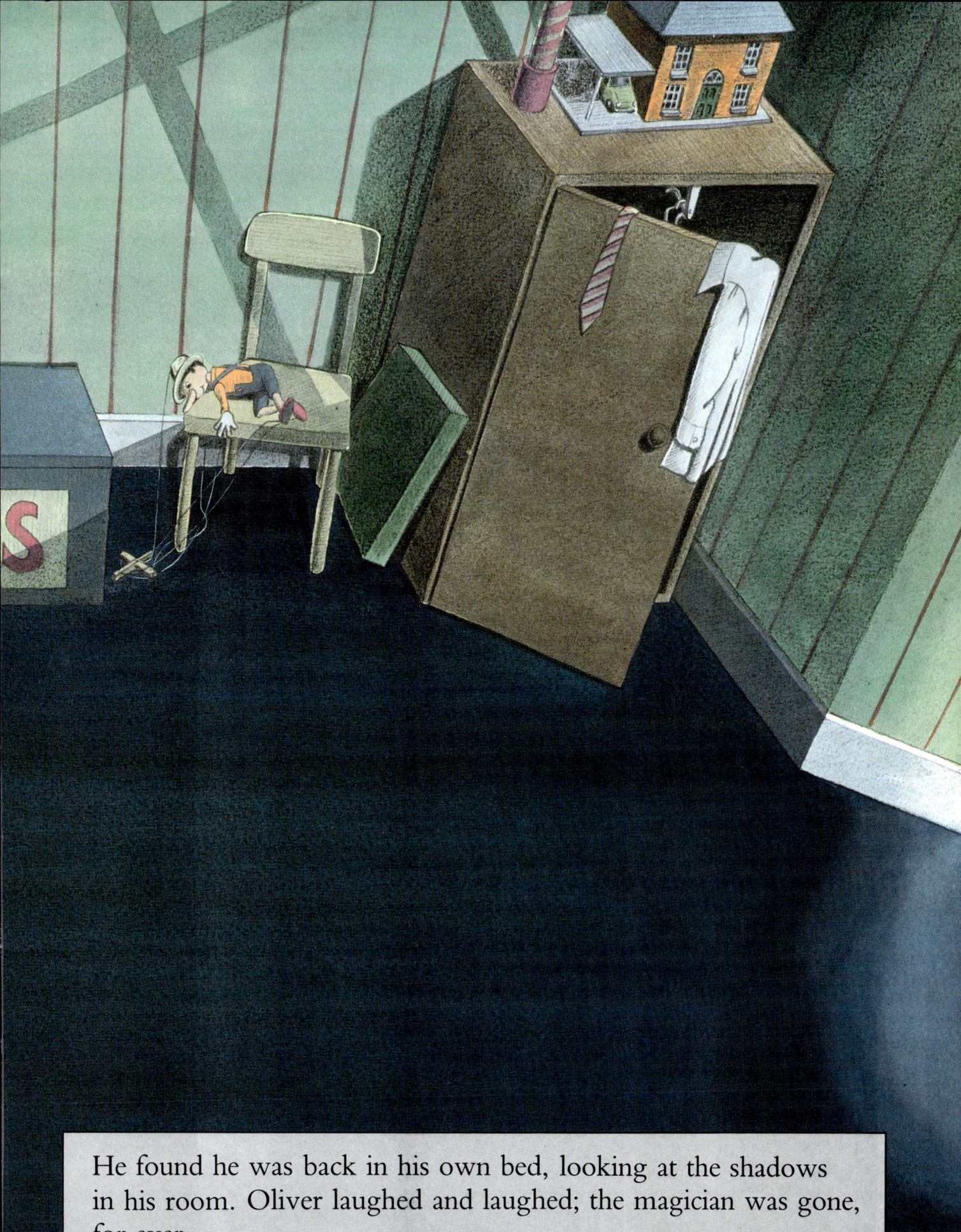

He found he was back in his own bed, looking at the shadows in his room. Oliver laughed and laughed; the magician was gone, for ever.

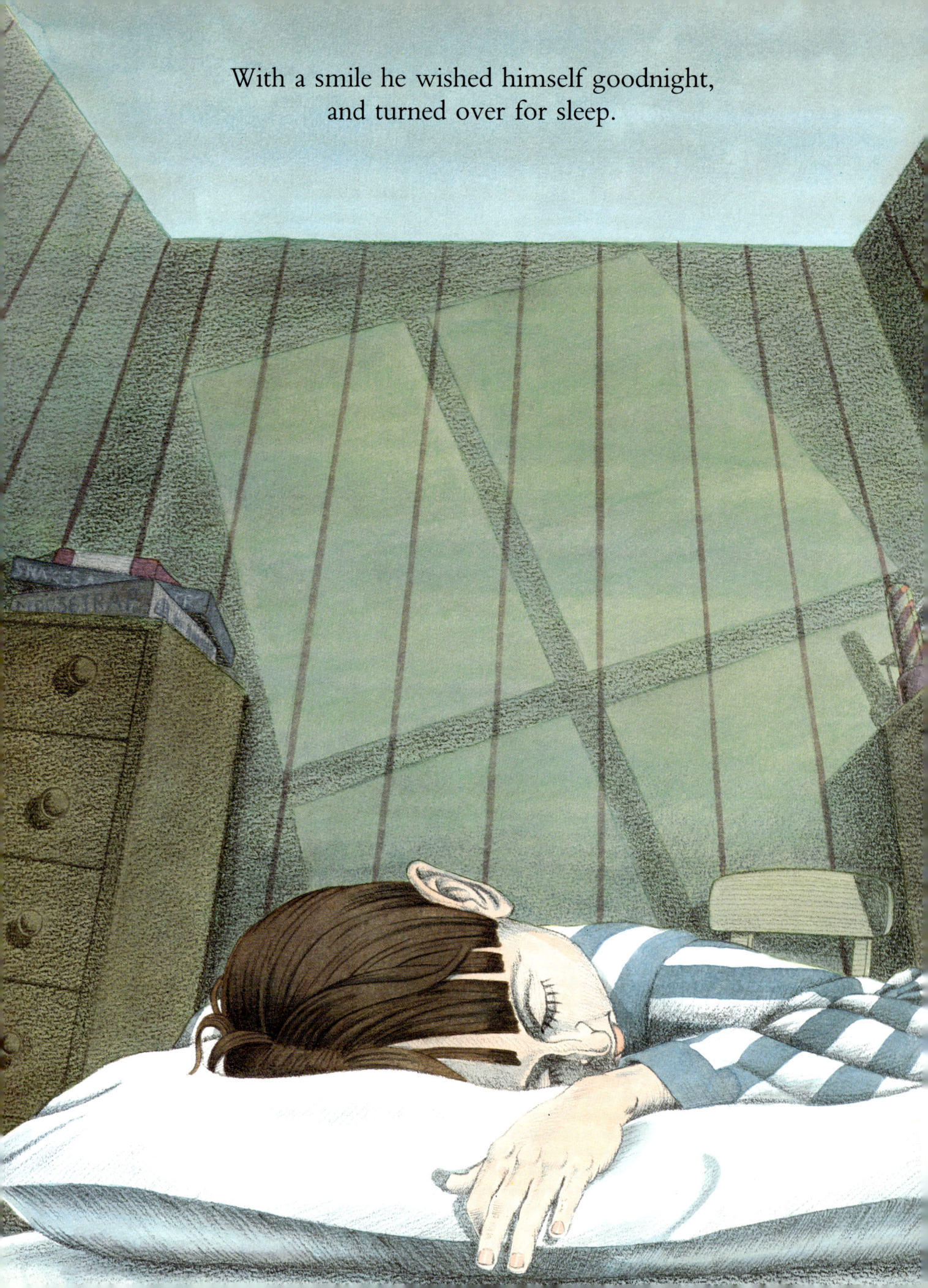